# A Comprehensive Guide to Choosing the Right Health Diet

* Balancing work, life, and diet.
* **4.3 Diet for Seniors**
  * Nutritional challenges of aging.
  * Importance of vitamins, minerals, and hydration.
* **4.4 Diet for Pregnant and Breastfeeding Women**
  * Nutritional needs for mother and baby.
  * Foods to prioritize and avoid.

## Chapter 5: Addressing Specific Health Conditions with Diet

* **5.1 Diet for Diabetes**
  * Managing blood sugar levels through diet.
  * Low glycemic index foods and portion control.
* **5.2 Diet for Hypertension**
  * Foods that help lower blood pressure.
  * The DASH diet and its benefits.
* **5.3 Diet for Autoimmune Diseases**
  * Anti-inflammatory diets and their impact.
  * The role of diet in managing symptoms.
* **5.4 Diet for Cancer Prevention and Support**
  * Nutritional strategies to reduce cancer risk.
  * Supporting the body during cancer treatment.
* **5.5 Diet for Osteoporosis**
  * Importance of calcium and vitamin D.
  * Foods and lifestyle habits to strengthen bones.

## Chapter 6: Practical Steps to Implementing a Healthy Diet

* **6.1 Setting Realistic Dietary Goals**
  * How to set achievable goals.
  * Tracking progress and staying motivated.
* **6.2 Meal Planning and Preparation**
  * Tips for effective meal planning.
  * How to prep meals for the week.
* **6.3 Grocery Shopping for a Healthy Diet**
  * Reading labels and choosing whole foods.
  * Tips for budget-friendly healthy shopping.

---

# Introduction

### 1.1 Understanding the Importance of Diet in Health

A healthy diet is the cornerstone of good health, directly influencing every aspect of our physical and mental well-being. What we eat provides the essential nutrients our bodies need to function correctly, maintain energy levels, and support growth and repair. Beyond basic sustenance, diet plays a critical role in preventing chronic diseases such as heart disease, diabetes, and certain cancers. The foods we choose also impact our mental health, affecting mood, cognition, and stress levels.

In the past century, there has been a dramatic shift in dietary patterns, primarily due to industrialization, globalization, and technological advancements. The rise of processed foods, fast food, and sugary beverages has led to an increase in diet-related health issues. Obesity rates have skyrocketed, and conditions like type 2 diabetes, cardiovascular diseases, and certain cancers have become more prevalent. Understanding the link between diet and health is essential for making informed decisions about what we eat.

A healthy diet is not a one-size-fits-all concept. It varies depending on individual needs, health conditions, and lifestyle factors. However, the foundation of a healthy diet remains consistent: a balance of macronutrients (carbohydrates, proteins, and fats), a variety of micronutrients (vitamins and minerals), adequate hydration, and moderation in the consumption of processed foods and sugars.

This guide is designed to help you navigate the complex world of nutrition and find a diet that suits your health goals, whether you want to lose weight, gain muscle, manage a chronic condition, or simply feel better overall. We'll explore various dietary approaches, break down the science of nutrition, and provide practical tips for implementing a healthy diet in your daily life.

## 1.2 Defining a "Healthy Diet"

The term "healthy diet" often conjures images of salads, green smoothies, and the elimination of all indulgences. However, a healthy diet is much more than a list of "good" and "bad" foods. It is about balance, variety, and moderation. A truly healthy diet is one that meets your nutritional needs, supports your physical and mental well-being, and is sustainable in the long term.

**Components of a Healthy Diet:**

- **Variety:** Eating a wide range of foods ensures that you get a broad spectrum of nutrients. This includes fruits, vegetables, whole grains, lean proteins, and healthy fats.
- **Balance:** Each meal should contain a balance of macronutrients—carbohydrates, proteins, and fats—tailored to your energy needs and health goals.
- **Moderation:** Portion control and moderation are crucial to avoid overeating, particularly with foods that are high in calories but low in nutrients, such as processed snacks and sugary drinks.
- **Nutrient Density:** Prioritize foods that are rich in vitamins, minerals, and other essential nutrients relative to their calorie content. This includes vegetables, fruits, lean proteins, and whole grains.
- **Hydration:** Adequate water intake is essential for all bodily functions, including digestion, nutrient absorption, and temperature regulation.

A healthy diet should also be flexible and enjoyable. It's not about strict limitations or depriving yourself of the foods you love. Instead, it's about making informed choices that contribute to your health while still allowing for occasional indulgences. The goal is to create a diet that you can maintain long-term, one that promotes overall health and well-being.

Throughout this guide, we will delve into various aspects of a healthy diet, from understanding the nutrients your body needs to exploring popular diet types and how to choose the right one for your health goals. Whether you're looking to improve your diet for weight management, enhance your fitness, or address specific health conditions, this guide will provide the knowledge and tools you need to make informed dietary choices.

# Chapter 1: The Science of Nutrition

## 1.1 Macronutrients: The Building Blocks of Diet

Macronutrients are the primary nutrients that our bodies need in large quantities to function correctly. They include carbohydrates, proteins, and fats, each playing a unique and vital role in maintaining health and energy levels.

### Carbohydrates: Types, Sources, and Functions

Carbohydrates are the body's primary source of energy. When consumed, they are broken down into glucose, which is then used by the body's cells for energy. There are two main types of carbohydrates: simple and complex.

- **Simple Carbohydrates:** These are sugars that provide a quick source of energy. They are found naturally in fruits, vegetables, and dairy products, but also in processed foods like candy, soda, and baked goods. While naturally occurring simple carbs are part of a healthy diet, added sugars should be consumed in moderation.
- **Complex Carbohydrates:** These include starches and fibers found in whole grains, legumes, and starchy vegetables like potatoes and corn. Complex carbohydrates are digested more slowly than simple carbs, providing a more sustained energy release. They also contain more nutrients and are usually higher in fiber, which is beneficial for digestive health.

The body needs carbohydrates for energy, brain function, and physical activity. The key to healthy carbohydrate consumption is focusing on whole, unprocessed sources that provide fiber, vitamins, and minerals.

### Proteins: Essential Amino Acids, Plant vs. Animal Sources

Proteins are essential for building and repairing tissues, producing enzymes and hormones, and supporting immune function. Proteins are made up of amino acids, which are categorized as either essential or non-essential. The body cannot produce essential amino acids, so they must be obtained from the diet.

- **Animal Proteins:** These are considered complete proteins because they contain all nine essential amino acids. Common sources include meat, poultry, fish, eggs, and dairy products.
- **Plant Proteins:** Most plant-based proteins are incomplete, meaning they lack one or more essential amino acids. However, by eating a variety of plant-based foods, such as beans, lentils, nuts, seeds, and whole grains, you can obtain all the essential amino acids. Some plant proteins, like quinoa and soy, are complete.

A balanced diet should include a mix of both plant and animal proteins to ensure a full spectrum of amino acids and other nutrients.

**Fats: Healthy vs. Unhealthy Fats, Role in the Body**

Fats are a critical component of a healthy diet, necessary for energy storage, cell structure, and the absorption of fat-soluble vitamins (A, D, E, and K). However, not all fats are created equal.

- **Unsaturated Fats:** These are considered the healthiest fats and include monounsaturated and polyunsaturated fats. Sources include olive oil, avocados, nuts, seeds, and fatty fish like salmon. Unsaturated fats are beneficial for heart health and can help reduce inflammation.
- **Saturated Fats:** Found in animal products like meat and dairy, as well as tropical oils like coconut oil, saturated fats should be consumed in moderation. Excessive intake can lead to increased cholesterol levels and a higher risk of heart disease.
- **Trans Fats:** These are the most harmful fats, often found in processed foods, baked goods, and fried foods. Trans fats can increase bad cholesterol levels (LDL) and decrease good cholesterol levels (HDL), significantly raising the risk of heart disease.

The key to fat consumption is moderation and choosing healthy sources. Replacing saturated and trans fats with unsaturated fats can have significant benefits for heart health.

## 1.2 Micronutrients: Vitamins and Minerals

Micronutrients, including vitamins and minerals, are required in smaller amounts than macronutrients but are just as vital for maintaining health. They play key roles in metabolic processes, immune function, and overall well-being.

**Essential Vitamins: Their Roles and Sources**

Vitamins are organic compounds that the body needs to perform various functions. They are categorized into two groups: water-soluble and fat-soluble.

- **Water-Soluble Vitamins:** These include the B-vitamins and vitamin C. They are not stored in the body and need to be consumed regularly. B-vitamins (like B12, B6, and folic acid) are crucial for energy production, brain function, and cell metabolism. Vitamin C is essential for immune function, skin health, and the absorption of iron.
    - **Sources:** Whole grains, fruits, vegetables, legumes, and animal products.
- **Fat-Soluble Vitamins:** These include vitamins A, D, E, and K, which are stored in the body's fatty tissues and liver. Vitamin A is essential for vision and immune function, vitamin D for bone health and immune support, vitamin E for its antioxidant properties, and vitamin K for blood clotting and bone metabolism.
    - **Sources:** Fatty fish, dairy products, eggs, leafy greens, and vegetable oils.

A diet rich in fruits, vegetables, whole grains, and healthy fats typically provides sufficient vitamins. However, some individuals may require supplements, particularly for vitamin D in areas with limited sunlight.

**Key Minerals: Importance and Dietary Sources**

Minerals are inorganic elements that play critical roles in bone health, nerve function, muscle contraction, and fluid balance. The most important minerals include calcium, potassium, magnesium, and iron.

- **Calcium:** Essential for strong bones and teeth, as well as muscle function and nerve transmission. Found in dairy products, leafy greens, and fortified foods.
- **Potassium:** Helps regulate fluid balance, muscle contractions, and nerve signals. High potassium intake can help reduce blood pressure and water retention. Sources include bananas, potatoes, beans, and fish.
- **Magnesium:** Supports muscle and nerve function, energy production, and bone health. Found in nuts, seeds, whole grains, and green leafy vegetables.
- **Iron:** Vital for the production of hemoglobin, which carries oxygen in the blood. Iron deficiency can lead to anemia. Sources include red meat, poultry, seafood, beans, and fortified cereals.

Adequate mineral intake is crucial for maintaining health, and deficiencies or excesses can lead to various health problems.

## 1.3 The Role of Water and Hydration

Water is essential for life, making up about 60% of the human body. It plays a crucial role in every bodily function, from regulating temperature and removing waste to lubricating joints and aiding digestion.

**Importance of Staying Hydrated**

Proper hydration is essential for maintaining the body's fluid balance, which is necessary for processes like circulation, digestion, and temperature regulation. Dehydration can lead to a range of health issues, including headaches, kidney stones, urinary tract infections, and impaired cognitive function.

**Daily Water Needs and the Impact of Hydration on Health**

The amount of water an individual needs varies depending on factors like age, weight, climate, and physical activity level. However, a general guideline is to drink about 8 cups (64 ounces) of water per day, though some people may need more. Hydration needs can also be met through the consumption of water-rich foods like fruits and vegetables.

Water plays a role in energy levels, physical performance, and overall health. Even mild dehydration can negatively affect mood and cognitive performance. It's crucial to drink water regularly throughout the day, especially during hot weather or periods of intense physical activity.

# Chapter 2: Popular Diet Types and Their Benefits

## 2.1 Overview of Common Diets

In today's health-conscious world, numerous diet types cater to different goals, lifestyles, and preferences. Understanding the principles, benefits, and potential drawbacks of these diets is crucial to making an informed choice that aligns with your health goals.

Diets can generally be categorized based on their primary focus, such as macronutrient ratios (e.g., low-carb vs. low-fat), the inclusion or exclusion of certain food groups (e.g., plant-based vs. animal-based), and meal timing (e.g., intermittent fasting). This chapter will explore some of the most popular and scientifically supported diets, providing insights into their benefits and who they might be best suited for.

## 2.2 The Mediterranean Diet

### Principles and Health Benefits

The Mediterranean diet is inspired by the traditional dietary patterns of countries bordering the Mediterranean Sea, particularly Greece, Italy, and Spain. It emphasizes whole, minimally processed foods, including:

- **Fruits and Vegetables:** A wide variety, including leafy greens, tomatoes, olives, and fruits like grapes and citrus.
- **Whole Grains:** Whole wheat, oats, barley, and other grains that provide fiber and essential nutrients.
- **Healthy Fats:** Olive oil as the primary source of fat, along with nuts, seeds, and avocados.
- **Lean Proteins:** Fish and seafood are prioritized over red meat, with moderate consumption of poultry, eggs, and dairy.
- **Herbs and Spices:** Used generously to flavor food, reducing the need for salt.
- **Moderate Alcohol Consumption:** Typically red wine, enjoyed with meals.

### Health Benefits

The Mediterranean diet is widely recognized for its heart health benefits, attributed to its emphasis on healthy fats, fiber, and antioxidants. Studies have shown that this diet can reduce the risk of cardiovascular diseases, lower cholesterol levels, and improve overall longevity. Additionally, it's associated with a lower incidence of certain cancers, diabetes, and neurodegenerative diseases like Alzheimer's.

### Foods to Include and Avoid

### To Include:

- Olive oil, nuts, seeds
- Whole grains, legumes
- Fresh fruits and vegetables
- Fish and seafood
- Moderate amounts of dairy (preferably fermented, like yogurt)
- Red wine in moderation

**To Avoid:**

- Processed foods
- Refined grains and sugars
- Excessive red meat and processed meats
- Butter and other animal fats (in large quantities)

The Mediterranean diet is particularly suitable for those looking for a sustainable, heart-healthy eating plan that doesn't require strict restrictions.

## 2.3 The Ketogenic Diet

### How It Works and Who It Benefits

The ketogenic (keto) diet is a high-fat, low-carbohydrate diet that shifts the body's metabolism from burning glucose (carbohydrates) to burning ketones (fats) for energy. This metabolic state is known as ketosis. The standard keto diet typically consists of:

- **70-75% Fat:** Healthy fats like avocados, nuts, seeds, olive oil, and butter.
- **20-25% Protein:** Moderate amounts of protein from sources like meat, fish, eggs, and dairy.
- **5-10% Carbohydrates:** Very low carb intake, primarily from non-starchy vegetables like leafy greens and cruciferous vegetables.

### Health Benefits

The keto diet has gained popularity for its effectiveness in weight loss, particularly for those struggling with obesity and insulin resistance. By significantly reducing carbohydrate intake, the body is forced to use fat as its primary energy source, leading to fat loss.

The keto diet has also been used therapeutically for neurological conditions like epilepsy, where it has been shown to reduce seizure frequency. Emerging research suggests potential benefits for other conditions, such as type 2 diabetes, metabolic syndrome, and certain cancers, although more studies are needed.

### Potential Risks and Long-Term Effects

While the keto diet can be effective for weight loss and certain health conditions, it's not without risks. Common side effects include the "keto flu," characterized by fatigue, headache, and nausea as the body adapts to ketosis. Long-term adherence to the keto diet may also lead to nutrient deficiencies, particularly in fiber, vitamins, and minerals found in fruits, vegetables, and whole grains.

The high fat intake, especially if it includes saturated fats, could potentially increase cholesterol levels and the risk of cardiovascular disease, although this is still debated in the scientific community.

The keto diet is best suited for those with specific health goals, such as rapid weight loss or managing epilepsy, and should be undertaken with medical supervision.

## 2.4 Plant-Based Diets (Vegan, Vegetarian)

### Nutritional Considerations and Benefits

Plant-based diets focus on foods derived from plants, including fruits, vegetables, nuts, seeds, oils, whole grains, legumes, and beans. There are variations within plant-based diets:

- **Vegan Diet:** Excludes all animal products, including meat, dairy, eggs, and often honey.
- **Vegetarian Diet:** Excludes meat, but may include dairy and eggs, depending on the type (e.g., lacto-vegetarian, ovo-vegetarian, lacto-ovo-vegetarian).

### Health Benefits

Plant-based diets are rich in fiber, vitamins, minerals, and antioxidants, all of which contribute to lower risks of chronic diseases such as heart disease, hypertension, type 2 diabetes, and certain cancers. They are also associated with lower body weight and improved digestive health due to high fiber intake.

### Nutritional Considerations

While plant-based diets offer many health benefits, they require careful planning to ensure nutritional adequacy. Vegans, in particular, need to be mindful of obtaining sufficient:

- **Protein:** From legumes, beans, tofu, tempeh, quinoa, and nuts.
- **Vitamin B12:** Which is not naturally found in plant foods, so supplementation or fortified foods are necessary.
- **Iron:** Non-heme iron from plants is less bioavailable, so combining it with vitamin C-rich foods can enhance absorption.
- **Calcium and Vitamin D:** Often sourced from fortified plant milks, leafy greens, and supplements.

- **Omega-3 Fatty Acids:** Can be obtained from flaxseeds, chia seeds, hemp seeds, and algae-based supplements.

A well-planned plant-based diet can provide all essential nutrients and is suitable for people at all stages of life, including pregnancy and infancy.

## 2.5 Paleo Diet

### Overview and Health Implications

The Paleo diet, also known as the "caveman" diet, is based on the premise of eating foods that were available to our hunter-gatherer ancestors. It emphasizes whole, unprocessed foods and excludes grains, legumes, dairy, and processed sugars. The diet primarily consists of:

- **Lean Meats:** Grass-fed beef, poultry, pork, and game meats.
- **Fish and Seafood:** Particularly those rich in omega-3 fatty acids.
- **Fruits and Vegetables:** Wide variety, particularly non-starchy vegetables.
- **Nuts and Seeds:** Except for legumes like peanuts.
- **Healthy Fats:** From avocados, nuts, seeds, and olive oil.

### Health Benefits

Proponents of the Paleo diet argue that it aligns more closely with human evolutionary needs and can reduce the risk of chronic diseases associated with modern diets. Benefits include improved blood sugar control, better satiety, weight loss, and reduced inflammation.

### Criticisms and Suitability

Critics of the Paleo diet point out that it excludes entire food groups, which can lead to nutrient deficiencies, particularly in calcium and vitamin D. The exclusion of grains and legumes also limits fiber intake, which is crucial for digestive health. Additionally, the emphasis on meat can raise concerns about saturated fat intake and environmental sustainability.

The Paleo diet may be suitable for individuals who prefer a high-protein, lower-carbohydrate diet and are not concerned with excluding dairy, grains, and legumes. However, it requires careful planning to ensure nutritional balance.

## 2.6 Low-Carb and Low-Fat Diets

### Comparison and Effectiveness

Low-carb and low-fat diets have been popular for decades, particularly for weight loss. Both approaches focus on macronutrient manipulation to achieve specific health outcomes.

### Low-Carb Diets:

- These diets reduce carbohydrate intake, often to less than 20% of total daily calories.
- Emphasize protein and fat consumption to promote satiety and fat burning.
- Common examples include the Atkins diet and the ketogenic diet.

**Low-Fat Diets:**

- These diets limit fat intake, typically to less than 30% of total daily calories.
- Focus on high-carbohydrate foods, particularly from whole grains, fruits, and vegetables.
- Common examples include the Ornish diet and traditional low-fat diets from the 1980s and 1990s.

**Which to Choose Based on Health Goals**

Both low-carb and low-fat diets can be effective for weight loss, but their success depends on individual factors such as metabolism, activity level, and personal preference.

- **Low-Carb Diets:** Often more effective for rapid weight loss, improving blood sugar control, and reducing insulin resistance. They may be more suitable for individuals with type 2 diabetes or metabolic syndrome.
- **Low-Fat Diets:** Can be effective for weight loss, particularly when combined with calorie restriction. They may be more suitable for those with a history of heart disease or high cholesterol levels, as they emphasize reducing saturated fat intake.

The best diet often depends on which approach is more sustainable for the individual. Long-term success relies on adherence and finding a balance that fits the person's lifestyle.

## 2.7 Fasting and Intermittent Fasting

**How Fasting Works**

Fasting is the practice of voluntarily abstaining from food for a specific period. Intermittent fasting (IF) has gained popularity as a dietary strategy for weight loss, metabolic health, and longevity. There are several methods of intermittent fasting, including:

- **16/8 Method:** Fasting for 16 hours and eating all meals within an 8-hour window.
- **5:2 Method:** Eating normally for five days a week and restricting calories (usually around 500-600 calories) for two non-consecutive days.
- **Eat-Stop-Eat:** Fasting for 24 hours once or twice a week.

**Health Benefits**

Intermittent fasting has been shown to have several potential health benefits, including:

- **Weight Loss:** By reducing the eating window, IF can help reduce overall calorie intake, leading to weight loss.

- **Improved Insulin Sensitivity:** Fasting periods allow insulin levels to decrease, which can improve insulin sensitivity and reduce the risk of type 2 diabetes.
- **Enhanced Cellular Repair:** Fasting triggers autophagy, a process where the body removes damaged cells and regenerates new ones, which may contribute to longevity and disease prevention.

**Potential Risks**

Fasting is not suitable for everyone, particularly individuals with a history of eating disorders, certain medical conditions, or those who are pregnant or breastfeeding. It can also lead to side effects like irritability, fatigue, and headaches, particularly during the adaptation period.

Intermittent fasting can be a powerful tool for weight management and metabolic health, but it should be approached with caution and tailored to individual needs.

## 2.8 Specialized Diets (Gluten-Free, Dairy-Free, etc.)

### Who Needs Them and Why

Specialized diets are designed for individuals with specific health conditions or intolerances that require the exclusion of certain foods. Common specialized diets include:

- **Gluten-Free Diet:** Necessary for individuals with celiac disease or non-celiac gluten sensitivity. Gluten is a protein found in wheat, barley, and rye, and avoiding it requires eliminating many processed foods and grains.
- **Dairy-Free Diet:** Required for those with lactose intolerance or a dairy allergy. This diet excludes all forms of dairy, including milk, cheese, yogurt, and butter.
- **Low-FODMAP Diet:** Used to manage irritable bowel syndrome (IBS) and other digestive disorders. It involves avoiding certain fermentable carbohydrates (FODMAPs) that can cause bloating, gas, and discomfort.

### Nutritional Challenges and Solutions

Specialized diets often come with nutritional challenges due to the exclusion of certain food groups. For example:

- **Gluten-Free Diet:** Can lead to a deficiency in fiber, iron, and B-vitamins typically found in fortified bread and cereals. Solutions include incorporating gluten-free whole grains like quinoa, brown rice, and buckwheat, and using fortified gluten-free products.

- **Dairy-Free Diet:** May result in insufficient calcium and vitamin D intake. Solutions include using fortified plant milks (like almond or soy milk), leafy greens, and supplements if necessary.
- **Low-FODMAP Diet:** Can be restrictive and may lead to inadequate fiber intake. Solutions include careful planning to ensure a variety of low-FODMAP fruits, vegetables, and grains are included.

Specialized diets require careful planning to ensure they meet all nutritional needs. Consulting with a healthcare provider or dietitian is often recommended for those starting a specialized diet.

## Chapter 3: Choosing the Right Diet for Your Health Goals

### 3.1 Understanding Personal Health Goals

Choosing the right diet is deeply personal and should align with your specific health goals. Whether your aim is weight loss, muscle gain, improved cardiovascular health, enhanced mental clarity, or managing a chronic condition, understanding your objectives will help you select the most effective dietary approach.

### Identifying Individual Needs and Goals

Before embarking on any diet, it's crucial to clearly define your health goals. These might include:

- **Weight Management:** Whether you want to lose, gain, or maintain your weight, your diet will play a pivotal role in achieving this.
- **Muscle Gain and Fitness:** For those looking to build muscle, a diet high in protein and adequate calories is essential.
- **Cardiovascular Health:** Diets focused on heart health typically emphasize reducing saturated fats, cholesterol, and sodium while increasing fiber and healthy fats.
- **Blood Sugar Control:** For managing diabetes or pre-diabetes, diets that stabilize blood sugar levels are crucial.
- **Digestive Health:** Some individuals may need to focus on diets that alleviate digestive issues, such as those with IBS or gluten intolerance.
- **Mental Well-being:** Nutrition has a profound impact on mental health, with certain diets helping to improve mood, cognitive function, and overall mental clarity.

Understanding your health goals will guide you in choosing the most suitable diet, ensuring it meets your nutritional needs and supports your overall well-being.

**How Lifestyle Factors Influence Diet Choice**

Your lifestyle plays a significant role in determining which diet is right for you. Consider the following factors:

- **Activity Level:** Highly active individuals, such as athletes, require more calories and specific nutrients like protein and carbohydrates to support their energy needs and muscle recovery.
- **Time Constraints:** Busy schedules might necessitate a diet that is easy to prepare and maintain, such as meal-prepped or simple whole-food-based diets.
- **Cultural and Ethical Considerations:** Cultural traditions and personal ethics (such as vegetarianism or veganism) will influence your diet choice.
- **Health Conditions:** Pre-existing health conditions, such as hypertension, diabetes, or food allergies, must be considered when choosing a diet.
- **Budget:** Some diets, like those emphasizing organic or specialty foods, can be more expensive. It's important to choose a diet that fits within your financial means.

By taking these factors into account, you can select a diet that not only meets your health goals but also integrates seamlessly into your lifestyle.

## 3.2 Diet for Weight Loss

Weight loss is one of the most common health goals, and numerous diets claim to be the best for shedding pounds. However, the most effective weight loss diets are those that promote sustainable, long-term results rather than quick fixes.

**How Different Diets Impact Weight Loss**

Various diets can lead to weight loss by creating a calorie deficit—where you consume fewer calories than your body needs to maintain its current weight. Here's how some popular diets approach weight loss:

- **Low-Carb Diets (e.g., Keto, Atkins):** These diets reduce carbohydrate intake, which lowers insulin levels and shifts the body's metabolism towards burning fat for energy. They can be particularly effective for those with insulin resistance or type 2 diabetes.
- **Low-Fat Diets:** These diets reduce fat intake, often leading to lower calorie consumption since fats are calorie-dense. Low-fat diets often focus on whole grains, fruits, and vegetables.
- **Intermittent Fasting:** This approach doesn't restrict specific foods but focuses on when you eat. By narrowing your eating window, you naturally reduce calorie intake, which can lead to weight loss.
- **Calorie Counting:** Some individuals find success by tracking their daily calorie intake to ensure they're consuming less than they burn. This method can be combined with any type of diet.

**Sustainable Practices for Long-Term Results**

The key to successful weight loss is sustainability. Extreme diets that drastically reduce calories or eliminate entire food groups may lead to quick weight loss but are often difficult to maintain long-term, leading to weight regain. Sustainable weight loss strategies include:

- **Moderation:** Focus on portion control rather than elimination of favorite foods. This helps in maintaining the diet over time.
- **Balanced Nutrition:** Ensure that your diet is balanced, providing all the essential nutrients your body needs to function optimally.
- **Behavioral Changes:** Adopt healthy habits such as mindful eating, regular physical activity, and adequate sleep to support weight loss.
- **Slow and Steady Approach:** Aim for a gradual weight loss of 1-2 pounds per week, which is more likely to be maintained in the long term.

By choosing a weight loss plan that aligns with your lifestyle and preferences, you can achieve lasting results without feeling deprived.

## 3.3 Diet for Muscle Gain and Fitness

Building muscle and improving fitness requires a diet that supports energy demands and provides the necessary nutrients for muscle repair and growth.

**Nutritional Strategies for Building Muscle**

To build muscle, you need to create a calorie surplus, meaning you consume more calories than you burn. However, it's not just about eating more; the quality of those calories matters too. Key strategies include:

- **High Protein Intake:** Protein is essential for muscle repair and growth. Aim for 1.2 to 2.2 grams of protein per kilogram of body weight, depending on your activity level and goals.
    - **Sources:** Lean meats, fish, eggs, dairy products, legumes, and plant-based protein sources like tofu and tempeh.
- **Sufficient Carbohydrates:** Carbs are your body's primary source of energy, especially during high-intensity workouts. Ensure you're getting enough complex carbohydrates to fuel your training.
    - **Sources:** Whole grains, fruits, vegetables, and legumes.
- **Healthy Fats:** Fats are crucial for hormone production, including testosterone, which plays a role in muscle growth. Include healthy fats in your diet to support overall health.
    - **Sources:** Avocados, nuts, seeds, and olive oil.

- **Timing and Frequency:** Eating frequent, balanced meals throughout the day ensures a steady supply of nutrients to your muscles. Pre- and post-workout nutrition are particularly important to optimize muscle repair and growth.

**Balancing Macros and Timing Meals**

Balancing macronutrients—protein, carbohydrates, and fats—is key to supporting muscle gain and fitness. A typical macro ratio for muscle building might be 40% carbohydrates, 30% protein, and 30% fat, but this can vary based on individual needs and preferences.

Meal timing is also crucial:

- **Pre-Workout:** Focus on carbs and protein to provide energy and prevent muscle breakdown. A small meal or snack 1-2 hours before training is ideal.
- **Post-Workout:** Consuming protein and carbs within 30-60 minutes after a workout helps replenish glycogen stores and kickstarts muscle repair. A protein shake or balanced meal is often recommended.

By focusing on nutrient timing and ensuring your diet supports your fitness goals, you can effectively build muscle and enhance overall performance.

### 3.4 Diet for Cardiovascular Health

Cardiovascular health is significantly influenced by diet. Certain foods can either increase or decrease the risk of heart disease, stroke, and other cardiovascular conditions.

**Nutrients That Support Heart Health**

A heart-healthy diet emphasizes nutrients that reduce inflammation, improve cholesterol levels, and lower blood pressure. Key nutrients include:

- **Fiber:** Helps reduce cholesterol levels by binding to cholesterol in the digestive system and promoting its excretion.
  - **Sources:** Whole grains, fruits, vegetables, and legumes.
- **Omega-3 Fatty Acids:** Reduce inflammation and lower the risk of heart disease by improving blood lipid levels and reducing blood pressure.
  - **Sources:** Fatty fish (like salmon, mackerel, and sardines), flaxseeds, chia seeds, and walnuts.
- **Antioxidants:** Protect against oxidative stress, which can damage the cardiovascular system.
  - **Sources:** Fruits and vegetables, particularly berries, citrus fruits, and leafy greens.
- **Magnesium and Potassium:** Help regulate blood pressure and support overall heart function.
  - **Sources:** Leafy greens, nuts, seeds, bananas, and avocados.

**Diets Proven to Reduce Cardiovascular Risk**

Several diets have been shown to be particularly effective in promoting heart health:

- **Mediterranean Diet:** Rich in fruits, vegetables, whole grains, and healthy fats, this diet has been linked to lower rates of heart disease.
- **DASH Diet (Dietary Approaches to Stop Hypertension):** Designed to lower blood pressure, the DASH diet emphasizes fruits, vegetables, whole grains, lean proteins, and low-fat dairy while limiting sodium, red meat, and sweets.
- **Plant-Based Diets:** Diets high in plant-based foods and low in animal products can reduce cholesterol levels and improve overall cardiovascular health.

For individuals concerned about heart health, adopting a diet that emphasizes these nutrients and dietary patterns can significantly reduce the risk of cardiovascular diseases.

## 3.5 Diet for Mental Health

The connection between diet and mental health is increasingly recognized, with research showing that certain nutrients can influence mood, cognition, and mental well-being.

**The Connection Between Diet and Mood**

What you eat can affect your brain function and emotional state. Diets rich in whole foods—particularly fruits, vegetables, whole grains, and lean proteins—are associated with better mental health outcomes. Key dietary factors include:

- **Omega-3 Fatty Acids:** Essential for brain health, omega-3s have been shown to reduce symptoms of depression and anxiety.
  - **Sources:** Fatty fish, flaxseeds, chia seeds, and walnuts.
- **Complex Carbohydrates:** Stabilize blood sugar levels, providing a steady supply of glucose to the brain and preventing mood swings.
  - **Sources:** Whole grains, legumes, and starchy vegetables.
- **Probiotics:** A healthy gut microbiome, supported by probiotics, has been linked to improved mood and reduced symptoms of anxiety and depression.
  - **Sources:** Yogurt, kefir, sauerkraut, and other fermented foods.
- **B-Vitamins:** Particularly B6, B12, and folate, which play a role in the production of neurotransmitters like serotonin.
  - **Sources:** Leafy greens, whole grains, eggs, and fortified cereals.

**Nutrients That Support Brain Function and Mental Well-being**

To support optimal mental health, focus on a diet that includes:

- **Antioxidant-Rich Foods:** Protect brain cells from oxidative stress, which can contribute to cognitive decline.
    - **Sources:** Berries, dark chocolate, nuts, and seeds.
- **Magnesium:** Known as the "relaxation mineral," magnesium helps regulate mood and improve sleep quality.
    - **Sources:** Leafy greens, nuts, seeds, and whole grains.
- **Tryptophan:** An amino acid that is a precursor to serotonin, which regulates mood.
    - **Sources:** Turkey, eggs, cheese, nuts, and seeds.

Adopting a diet rich in these nutrients can help improve mental clarity, reduce symptoms of depression and anxiety, and enhance overall emotional well-being.

### 3.6 Diet for Digestive Health

Digestive health is crucial for overall well-being, as it affects nutrient absorption, immune function, and even mental health. Dietary choices can either promote or impair digestive function.

### Common Digestive Issues and Dietary Solutions

Digestive problems like bloating, constipation, diarrhea, and acid reflux are common, but diet can play a significant role in managing these conditions:

- **High-Fiber Diet:** Increasing fiber intake is key for preventing constipation and promoting regular bowel movements. Both soluble and insoluble fiber are important.
    - **Sources:** Whole grains, fruits, vegetables, legumes, and nuts.

- **Probiotic-Rich Foods:** Probiotics support a healthy gut microbiome, which is essential for digestion and immunity.
    - **Sources:** Yogurt, kefir, kimchi, sauerkraut, and other fermented foods.
- **Low-FODMAP Diet:** For those with IBS, reducing intake of fermentable oligosaccharides, disaccharides, monosaccharides, and polyols (FODMAPs) can alleviate symptoms.
    - **Sources to Reduce:** Onions, garlic, beans, certain fruits, and artificial sweeteners.
- **Hydration:** Adequate water intake is essential for preventing constipation and supporting overall digestive health.

### The Role of Fiber, Probiotics, and Hydration

Fiber, probiotics, and hydration are the cornerstones of a healthy digestive system:

- **Fiber:** Helps maintain bowel regularity, prevent constipation, and feed beneficial gut bacteria.

- **Probiotics:** Balance the gut microbiome, supporting digestion and immunity.
- **Hydration:** Keeps the digestive system running smoothly by aiding in the digestion and absorption of nutrients.

For individuals experiencing digestive issues, focusing on these aspects of diet can help improve gut health and overall well-being.

# Chapter 4: Tailoring Diets to Different Life Stages

## 4.1 Diet for Children and Adolescents

Nutritional needs vary significantly throughout different stages of life, starting from childhood through adolescence. Proper nutrition during these critical growth periods sets the foundation for lifelong health and well-being.

### Nutritional Needs During Growth

Children and adolescents have higher nutritional demands than adults because they are growing and developing at a rapid pace. Key nutrients required for this growth include:

- **Protein:** Essential for growth, tissue repair, and immune function. Children need adequate protein to support their developing muscles, organs, and bones.
  - **Sources:** Lean meats, fish, eggs, dairy, beans, and legumes.
- **Calcium and Vitamin D:** Critical for bone development. Adequate calcium intake is essential for building strong bones, while vitamin D aids calcium absorption.
  - **Sources:** Dairy products, fortified plant milks, leafy greens, and sunlight exposure (for vitamin D).
- **Iron:** Necessary for cognitive development and the production of hemoglobin, which carries oxygen in the blood. Adolescents, particularly girls, need to ensure they get enough iron to support growth and prevent anemia.
  - **Sources:** Red meat, poultry, beans, lentils, and fortified cereals.
- **Healthy Fats:** Support brain development and overall energy needs. Omega-3 fatty acids, in particular, are vital for cognitive function and eye health.
  - **Sources:** Fatty fish, nuts, seeds, and avocados.
- **Vitamins and Minerals:** A variety of vitamins and minerals are necessary for overall health, including vitamins A, C, E, and zinc, which support immune function and healthy skin.

### Addressing Picky Eating and Balanced Meals

Many children are picky eaters, which can make it challenging to ensure they receive a balanced diet. Strategies to encourage healthy eating habits include:

- **Role Modeling:** Children are more likely to eat healthy foods if they see their parents and caregivers doing the same. Serve a variety of nutritious foods at family meals.

- **Involving Children in Food Preparation:** Letting children help with meal planning and cooking can increase their interest in trying new foods.
- **Offering a Variety of Foods:** Regularly introduce new fruits, vegetables, and whole grains alongside familiar favorites to expand their palate.
- **Making Healthy Foods Fun:** Presenting fruits and vegetables in fun shapes or as part of colorful meals can make them more appealing to children.
- **Consistent Mealtimes:** Having regular meal and snack times helps children develop a healthy relationship with food and reduces the likelihood of overeating.

Ensuring children and adolescents receive balanced meals with all essential nutrients will support their growth, development, and overall health.

## 4.2 Diet for Adults

As individuals transition into adulthood, their nutritional needs evolve. While the focus often shifts from growth to maintaining health, adults still require a balanced diet to support their energy needs, prevent chronic diseases, and sustain mental and physical well-being.

### Adjusting Diets as Metabolism Changes

As adults age, metabolism tends to slow down, leading to a decreased calorie requirement. This change means that dietary focus should shift towards nutrient-dense foods that provide essential vitamins and minerals without excessive calories. Key considerations include:

- **Portion Control:** With a slower metabolism, portion control becomes crucial to avoid weight gain. Smaller, more frequent meals can help regulate hunger and energy levels.
- **Balanced Macronutrients:** A balanced intake of carbohydrates, proteins, and fats remains important, but the type of each macronutrient should be carefully considered. For example, focusing on whole grains, lean proteins, and healthy fats can help maintain energy and prevent chronic conditions.
- **Increased Fiber Intake:** As metabolism slows, the digestive system may also become less efficient. Increasing fiber intake helps maintain digestive health and can aid in weight management.
  - **Sources:** Whole grains, fruits, vegetables, beans, and legumes.
- **Hydration:** Maintaining proper hydration is essential, as water needs don't decrease with age, but the body's ability to conserve water may diminish.

### Balancing Work, Life, and Diet

Busy adult lives often make it challenging to maintain a healthy diet. Strategies to balance work, life, and diet include:

- **Meal Planning:** Preparing meals in advance can save time and ensure that healthy options are always available. Batch cooking and meal prepping on weekends can reduce the temptation to eat out or rely on convenience foods during the week.
- **Healthy Snacking:** Keeping healthy snacks on hand, such as nuts, fruits, and yogurt, can help maintain energy levels throughout the day and prevent overeating at meals.
- **Mindful Eating:** Being mindful of eating habits, such as avoiding eating in front of the TV or at the desk, can help prevent overeating and improve digestion.
- **Stress Management:** Managing stress through exercise, meditation, and adequate sleep can reduce the likelihood of emotional eating and support overall health.

By adjusting dietary habits to fit a changing metabolism and busy lifestyle, adults can maintain optimal health and prevent the onset of diet-related conditions.

## 4.3 Diet for Seniors

As individuals enter their senior years, their nutritional needs change once again. A focus on nutrient-dense foods, adequate hydration, and proper digestion becomes increasingly important to maintain health and vitality.

## Nutritional Challenges of Aging

Aging can bring about several nutritional challenges, including decreased appetite, changes in taste and smell, and difficulty chewing or swallowing. Seniors may also have a reduced ability to absorb certain nutrients, making it essential to focus on nutrient-rich foods:

- **Calcium and Vitamin D:** As bone density decreases with age, it's crucial to get enough calcium and vitamin D to support bone health and prevent osteoporosis.
  - **Sources:** Fortified plant milks, leafy greens, and supplements.
- **B12 and Folate:** Absorption of vitamin B12 decreases with age, leading to a higher risk of deficiency, which can cause anemia and cognitive decline. Folate also supports cognitive function and heart health.
  - **Sources:** Fortified cereals, lean meats, and B12 supplements.
- **Protein:** Protein needs remain high in older adults to prevent muscle loss (sarcopenia) and support overall strength and mobility.
  - **Sources:** Lean meats, dairy products, beans, legumes, and protein-rich plant foods.
- **Fiber:** To prevent constipation and support digestive health, a diet high in fiber is recommended.
  - **Sources:** Whole grains, fruits, vegetables, and legumes.
- **Hydration:** Seniors are at a higher risk of dehydration due to a diminished sense of thirst. Ensuring adequate fluid intake is crucial for maintaining kidney function and overall health.

**Importance of Vitamins, Minerals, and Hydration**

Ensuring that seniors get enough essential vitamins and minerals is critical for preventing age-related health issues. Additionally, staying hydrated can prevent a range of problems, from constipation to urinary tract infections and kidney stones.

Seniors should focus on:

- **Nutrient-Dense Foods:** Choosing foods that are high in vitamins and minerals but low in calories can help meet nutritional needs without overeating.
- **Small, Frequent Meals:** If appetite is an issue, smaller, more frequent meals can help ensure adequate nutrient intake.
- **Hydration Reminders:** Encouraging regular fluid intake, even if not thirsty, can help prevent dehydration.

A balanced diet tailored to the unique needs of seniors can help maintain health, prevent chronic diseases, and support overall quality of life.

**4.4 Diet for Pregnant and Breastfeeding Women**

Pregnancy and breastfeeding are times of increased nutritional demands, as the body is supporting both the mother and the developing baby. Proper nutrition is essential for the health of both.

**Nutritional Needs for Mother and Baby**

During pregnancy and breastfeeding, certain nutrients become particularly important:

- **Folate (Vitamin B9):** Crucial for preventing neural tube defects in the developing baby. It's recommended that women of childbearing age consume 400-800 micrograms of folate daily, particularly before conception and during the first trimester.
  - **Sources:** Leafy greens, fortified cereals, legumes, and supplements.
- **Iron:** Supports the increased blood volume during pregnancy and prevents anemia. Iron needs double during pregnancy, making it essential to consume enough through diet and, if necessary, supplements.
  - **Sources:** Red meat, poultry, fish, beans, and fortified cereals.
- **Calcium and Vitamin D:** Essential for the development of the baby's bones and teeth. These nutrients also support the mother's bone health.
  - **Sources:** Dairy products, fortified plant milks, leafy greens, and supplements.

- **Omega-3 Fatty Acids:** Important for the baby's brain and eye development. DHA, a type of omega-3, is particularly critical.
    - **Sources:** Fatty fish, flaxseeds, chia seeds, and DHA supplements.
- **Protein:** Increased protein intake supports the growth of fetal tissues, including the brain, and helps in the production of breast milk.
    - **Sources:** Lean meats, poultry, fish, dairy products, beans, and legumes.
- **Hydration:** Adequate fluid intake is essential for maintaining amniotic fluid levels and supporting increased blood volume.

**Foods to Prioritize and Avoid**

Certain foods should be prioritized during pregnancy and breastfeeding to ensure both mother and baby receive the necessary nutrients. Conversely, some foods should be avoided to reduce the risk of foodborne illnesses and exposure to harmful substances:

**To Prioritize:**

- **Fruits and Vegetables:** Provide essential vitamins, minerals, and fiber.
- **Whole Grains:** Offer energy and important nutrients like iron and B-vitamins.
- **Lean Proteins:** Support the increased protein needs of pregnancy and breastfeeding.
- **Dairy or Fortified Plant Milks:** Provide calcium, vitamin D, and protein.
- **Healthy Fats:** Support the development of the baby's brain and nervous system.

**To Avoid:**

- **Raw or Undercooked Seafood and Eggs:** Pose a risk of foodborne illness, such as salmonella or listeria.
- **High-Mercury Fish:** Includes species like shark, swordfish, king mackerel, and tilefish, which can be harmful to the baby's developing nervous system.
- **Unpasteurized Dairy Products:** Risk of listeria infection.
- **Alcohol:** Should be avoided entirely during pregnancy due to the risk of fetal alcohol syndrome.
- **Excessive Caffeine:** High caffeine intake can increase the risk of miscarriage and low birth weight.

By focusing on a balanced diet that meets these increased nutritional demands, pregnant and breastfeeding women can support their health and the health of their baby.

# Chapter 5: Addressing Specific Health Conditions with Diet

## 5.1 Diet for Diabetes

Diabetes is a chronic condition characterized by elevated blood sugar levels. Managing diabetes effectively involves maintaining stable blood glucose levels through diet, physical activity, and sometimes medication. A well-planned diet is crucial in preventing complications and maintaining overall health.

### Managing Blood Sugar Levels Through Diet

For individuals with diabetes, the primary goal is to maintain blood sugar levels within a target range. Key dietary strategies include:

- **Carbohydrate Management:** Since carbohydrates have the most significant impact on blood sugar levels, managing the type and amount of carbohydrates consumed is essential. Focus on complex carbohydrates that have a lower glycemic index (GI).
  - **Sources:** Whole grains, legumes, fruits, and non-starchy vegetables.
- **Portion Control:** Eating smaller, balanced meals throughout the day can help prevent spikes and dips in blood sugar levels. Portion control is particularly important for carbohydrate-rich foods.
- **Glycemic Index Awareness:** The glycemic index measures how quickly a carbohydrate-containing food raises blood sugar levels. Foods with a lower GI are digested more slowly, resulting in a more gradual increase in blood glucose.
  - **Low-GI Foods:** Whole grains, legumes, non-starchy vegetables, and most fruits.
  - **High-GI Foods to Limit:** White bread, sugary cereals, potatoes, and sweetened beverages.
- **Fiber Intake:** Fiber slows the absorption of sugar into the bloodstream, which helps regulate blood sugar levels. A high-fiber diet can improve glycemic control and reduce the risk of heart disease.
  - **Sources:** Whole grains, fruits, vegetables, beans, and nuts.
- **Healthy Fats:** Incorporating healthy fats, such as those found in olive oil, avocados, and nuts, can help manage blood sugar levels and reduce the risk of cardiovascular complications.
- **Consistent Meal Timing:** Eating at regular intervals can help maintain stable blood sugar levels throughout the day.

### Low Glycemic Index Foods and Portion Control

A diabetes-friendly diet should emphasize low-GI foods and proper portion control. Examples of low-GI foods include:

- **Whole Grains:** Brown rice, quinoa, barley, and oats.

- **Legumes:** Lentils, chickpeas, and black beans.
- **Fruits:** Apples, pears, berries, and oranges.
- **Vegetables:** Leafy greens, broccoli, cauliflower, and carrots.

Portion control is also crucial, particularly for carbohydrate-rich foods. Using smaller plates, measuring portions, and paying attention to hunger cues can help maintain portion control and prevent overeating.

By focusing on these dietary strategies, individuals with diabetes can manage their blood sugar levels effectively and reduce the risk of complications.

### 5.2 Diet for Hypertension

Hypertension, or high blood pressure, is a common condition that increases the risk of heart disease, stroke, and other health problems. Diet plays a critical role in managing blood pressure, and certain dietary approaches have been proven effective in lowering and maintaining healthy blood pressure levels.

### Foods That Help Lower Blood Pressure

Several nutrients are particularly beneficial for lowering blood pressure, including potassium, magnesium, calcium, and dietary fiber. Key foods that support healthy blood pressure include:

- **Leafy Greens:** Rich in potassium, which helps balance sodium levels in the body, leafy greens like spinach, kale, and Swiss chard can help lower blood pressure.
- **Berries:** High in flavonoids, berries such as blueberries, strawberries, and raspberries have been shown to reduce blood pressure and improve heart health.
- **Beets:** Beets are high in nitrates, which help relax blood vessels and improve blood flow, thereby reducing blood pressure.
- **Oats:** Oats contain beta-glucan, a type of soluble fiber that has been shown to lower cholesterol and improve blood pressure.
- **Bananas:** Another potassium-rich food, bananas help manage blood pressure by counteracting the effects of sodium.
- **Garlic:** Garlic has been shown to have blood pressure-lowering effects due to its ability to increase nitric oxide in the body, which relaxes blood vessels.
- **Fish High in Omega-3s:** Fatty fish like salmon, mackerel, and sardines are rich in omega-3 fatty acids, which reduce inflammation and lower blood pressure.

### The DASH Diet and Its Benefits

The Dietary Approaches to Stop Hypertension (DASH) diet is specifically designed to prevent and control high blood pressure. The DASH diet emphasizes:

- **Fruits and Vegetables:** At least 4-5 servings of each per day.

- **Whole Grains:** 6-8 servings per day, focusing on fiber-rich options like whole wheat bread, brown rice, and oats.
- **Low-Fat Dairy Products:** 2-3 servings per day of milk, yogurt, or cheese.
- **Lean Proteins:** Emphasizing fish, poultry, beans, and nuts while limiting red meat.
- **Limiting Sodium:** Reducing sodium intake to 2,300 mg per day, or ideally, 1,500 mg per day for individuals with hypertension or higher risk.

The DASH diet has been extensively studied and shown to significantly lower blood pressure, reduce LDL cholesterol, and improve overall cardiovascular health. It's an effective and sustainable approach to managing hypertension.

## 5.3 Diet for Autoimmune Diseases

Autoimmune diseases occur when the immune system mistakenly attacks the body's tissues, leading to inflammation and a range of symptoms. While diet cannot cure autoimmune diseases, it can play a significant role in managing symptoms and reducing inflammation.

### Anti-inflammatory Diets and Their Impact

An anti-inflammatory diet focuses on foods that reduce inflammation and avoid those that may exacerbate it. Key components of an anti-inflammatory diet include:

- **Fruits and Vegetables:** Rich in antioxidants and phytochemicals, these foods help combat oxidative stress and inflammation.
  - **Examples:** Berries, leafy greens, cruciferous vegetables, and citrus fruits.
- **Healthy Fats:** Omega-3 fatty acids, in particular, have strong anti-inflammatory properties.
  - **Sources:** Fatty fish, flaxseeds, chia seeds, walnuts, and olive oil.
- **Whole Grains:** Whole grains provide fiber, which supports gut health and reduces inflammation.
  - **Examples:** Brown rice, quinoa, oats, and whole wheat.
- **Spices:** Certain spices, such as turmeric and ginger, have potent anti-inflammatory effects.
- **Probiotic-Rich Foods:** A healthy gut microbiome can modulate the immune response and reduce inflammation.
  - **Sources:** Yogurt, kefir, sauerkraut, kimchi, and other fermented foods.

### The Role of Diet in Managing Symptoms

For individuals with autoimmune diseases, diet can help manage symptoms by:

- **Reducing Inflammation:** An anti-inflammatory diet can reduce the frequency and severity of flare-ups.

- **Supporting Gut Health:** A healthy gut is crucial for immune regulation. Probiotic and fiber-rich foods support gut health, which may help modulate the immune system.
- **Avoiding Trigger Foods:** Some individuals with autoimmune diseases may have food sensitivities that trigger symptoms. Common triggers include gluten, dairy, and nightshade vegetables (tomatoes, peppers, potatoes, and eggplants). An elimination diet can help identify these triggers.

Managing autoimmune diseases often requires a personalized approach, as triggers and beneficial foods can vary between individuals. Consulting with a healthcare provider or dietitian can help tailor a diet that supports symptom management and overall health.

## 5.4 Diet for Cancer Prevention and Support

Diet plays a critical role in both the prevention and management of cancer. Certain foods can help reduce the risk of developing cancer, while others can support the body during treatment and recovery.

### Nutritional Strategies to Reduce Cancer Risk

A diet that supports cancer prevention emphasizes whole, nutrient-dense foods and minimizes exposure to potential carcinogens. Key dietary strategies include:

- **Fruits and Vegetables:** Rich in antioxidants, vitamins, and phytochemicals, fruits and vegetables help protect cells from damage that can lead to cancer. Cruciferous vegetables like broccoli, cauliflower, and Brussels sprouts are particularly beneficial.
- **Whole Grains:** High in fiber, whole grains support digestive health and may reduce the risk of colorectal cancer.
    - **Examples:** Brown rice, oats, quinoa, and whole wheat products.
- **Healthy Fats:** Omega-3 fatty acids, found in fatty fish, flaxseeds, and walnuts, have anti-inflammatory properties that may reduce cancer risk.
- **Limit Red and Processed Meats:** Studies have shown that high consumption of red and processed meats can increase the risk of colorectal and other cancers. Limiting these foods and focusing on plant-based proteins can be beneficial.
- **Avoiding Sugary Foods and Drinks:** Excess sugar intake is linked to obesity, a risk factor for several types of cancer. Reducing sugar intake can help maintain a healthy weight and lower cancer risk.
- **Moderate Alcohol Consumption:** Alcohol consumption is associated with an increased risk of several cancers, including breast and liver cancer. Limiting alcohol to moderate levels or avoiding it altogether is recommended.

### Supporting the Body During Cancer Treatment

Cancer treatment, including chemotherapy and radiation, can take a toll on the body, leading to side effects like nausea, loss of appetite, and weakened immunity. A supportive diet during treatment should focus on:

- **Nutrient-Dense Foods:** Since appetite may be reduced, it's important to consume foods that are rich in vitamins, minerals, and calories to meet nutritional needs.
    - **Examples:** Smoothies with fruits, vegetables, protein powders, and healthy fats.
- **Small, Frequent Meals:** Eating smaller, more frequent meals can help manage nausea and maintain energy levels.
- **Hydration:** Staying hydrated is crucial, particularly during treatment, as it helps manage side effects like dry mouth and fatigue.
- **Protein:** Adequate protein intake supports tissue repair and immune function during treatment.
    - **Sources:** Lean meats, fish, eggs, dairy, beans, and legumes.
- **Soft Foods:** If mouth sores or difficulty swallowing occur, soft foods like mashed potatoes, yogurt, and soups can be easier to eat.

A diet tailored to the individual's needs during cancer treatment can help manage side effects, maintain strength, and support recovery.

**5.5 Diet for Osteoporosis**

Osteoporosis is a condition characterized by weakened bones, increasing the risk of fractures. Diet plays a crucial role in maintaining bone density and preventing osteoporosis, particularly in postmenopausal women and older adults.

**Importance of Calcium and Vitamin D**

Calcium and vitamin D are the two most important nutrients for bone health:

- **Calcium:** Calcium is the primary mineral found in bones and is essential for maintaining bone strength and density. Adults need about 1,000 mg of calcium per day, with the requirement increasing to 1,200 mg for women over 50 and men over 70.
    - **Sources:** Dairy products, fortified plant milks, leafy greens, almonds, and calcium-fortified foods.
- **Vitamin D:** Vitamin D is crucial for calcium absorption and bone metabolism. Without adequate vitamin D, the body cannot absorb calcium effectively, leading to bone loss.
    - **Sources:** Sunlight exposure, fatty fish, fortified foods, and vitamin D supplements.

**Foods and Lifestyle Habits to Strengthen Bones**

In addition to calcium and vitamin D, several other nutrients and lifestyle habits contribute to bone health:

- **Protein:** Adequate protein intake is essential for bone health, as protein forms part of the bone matrix. However, it's important to balance protein intake with calcium-rich foods.
    - **Sources:** Lean meats, fish, dairy products, and plant-based proteins.
- **Magnesium and Potassium:** These minerals play a role in bone health by supporting calcium metabolism and reducing bone loss.
    - **Sources:** Leafy greens, nuts, seeds, bananas, and whole grains.
- **Vitamin K:** Vitamin K helps regulate calcium in the bones and supports bone formation.
    - **Sources:** Leafy greens, broccoli, and Brussels sprouts.
- **Avoiding Excess Sodium and Caffeine:** High sodium and caffeine intake can increase calcium excretion, which may weaken bones. Limiting these substances can help preserve bone density.
- **Weight-Bearing Exercise:** Regular physical activity, particularly weight-bearing exercises like walking, jogging, and strength training, is crucial for maintaining bone density and preventing osteoporosis.

By focusing on a diet rich in bone-supporting nutrients and incorporating regular exercise, individuals can maintain strong bones and reduce the risk of osteoporosis and fractures.

## Chapter 6: Practical Steps to Implementing a Healthy Diet

### 6.1 Setting Realistic Dietary Goals

Adopting a healthy diet is a journey that requires setting realistic, achievable goals. Clear and attainable goals provide direction and motivation, helping you stay on track and make lasting changes.

### How to Set Achievable Goals

When setting dietary goals, it's important to use the SMART criteria—goals should be Specific, Measurable, Achievable, Relevant, and Time-bound. Here's how to apply this framework:

- **Specific:** Clearly define what you want to achieve. For example, instead of saying "I want to eat healthier," specify that "I want to increase my intake of fruits and vegetables to five servings per day."
- **Measurable:** Ensure your goal is quantifiable so you can track your progress. For instance, "I will drink eight glasses of water a day" is a measurable goal.

- **Achievable:** Set goals that are challenging yet realistic. If you're currently eating out three times a week, reducing it to once a week might be more realistic than eliminating it entirely.
- **Relevant:** Your goals should align with your broader health objectives. If your aim is to lose weight, a relevant goal might be "I will reduce my intake of sugary drinks to only one per week."
- **Time-bound:** Set a deadline for your goals to create a sense of urgency and help you stay focused. For example, "I will achieve my goal of five servings of vegetables per day within three months."

## Tracking Progress and Staying Motivated

Monitoring your progress is crucial to achieving your dietary goals. Here are some strategies to help you stay on track:

- **Food Journals:** Keeping a food diary can help you track what you eat and identify patterns. You can use a physical journal or a digital app to log your meals, snacks, and beverages.
- **Regular Check-ins:** Set aside time each week to review your progress. Assess what's working, what challenges you're facing, and how you can adjust your goals or strategies.
- **Celebrate Milestones:** Recognize and celebrate small achievements along the way. This could be as simple as acknowledging that you've met your hydration goals for the week or that you've tried a new vegetable.
- **Stay Flexible:** Life is unpredictable, and it's important to be flexible with your goals. If you miss a day or fall off track, don't be discouraged—refocus and continue moving forward.

By setting realistic goals and regularly tracking your progress, you can build healthy eating habits that last a lifetime.

## 6.2 Meal Planning and Preparation

Meal planning and preparation are powerful tools for maintaining a healthy diet. By taking the time to plan your meals in advance, you can ensure that you're eating balanced, nutritious meals throughout the week, even on busy days.

## Tips for Effective Meal Planning

Effective meal planning involves selecting meals that meet your nutritional needs, are easy to prepare, and align with your lifestyle. Here's how to get started:

- **Plan for the Week Ahead:** Choose a day each week to plan your meals for the upcoming week. Consider your schedule, dietary goals, and any social events that may impact your meals.

- **Create a Balanced Menu:** Aim to include a variety of food groups in each meal—proteins, carbohydrates, healthy fats, and plenty of fruits and vegetables. This ensures you're getting all the necessary nutrients.
- **Incorporate Leftovers:** Plan meals that can be easily transformed into leftovers for the next day's lunch or dinner. This saves time and reduces food waste.
- **Prep Ingredients in Advance:** Chop vegetables, cook grains, and marinate proteins ahead of time to make meal preparation quicker during the week.
- **Consider Batch Cooking:** Prepare large quantities of certain dishes, like soups, stews, or casseroles, and freeze portions for future meals. This is especially helpful for busy days when you don't have time to cook.

**How to Prep Meals for the Week**

Meal prepping involves preparing multiple meals or ingredients ahead of time, making it easier to eat healthy throughout the week. Here's a step-by-step guide:

1. **Choose Recipes:** Select 3-4 recipes that you enjoy and that align with your dietary goals. Aim for a variety of proteins, vegetables, and whole grains.
2. **Grocery Shopping:** Make a list of the ingredients you need and do your grocery shopping for the week. Stick to your list to avoid impulse purchases.
3. **Batch Cooking:** Set aside a few hours on a designated day (like Sunday) to cook your meals. Prepare grains, proteins, and vegetables in bulk.


4. **Portion and Store:** Divide your meals into individual portions and store them in airtight containers. Label each container with the date and contents.
5. **Reheat and Enjoy:** Throughout the week, simply reheat your prepped meals as needed. You can mix and match components to keep meals varied and interesting.

Meal prepping saves time, reduces stress, and helps you stick to your dietary goals by ensuring you always have healthy options on hand.

**6.3 Grocery Shopping for a Healthy Diet**

Healthy eating starts with smart grocery shopping. By making informed choices at the grocery store, you can stock your kitchen with nutritious foods that support your dietary goals.

**Reading Labels and Choosing Whole Foods**

Understanding how to read food labels is essential for making healthy choices. Here's what to look for:

- **Ingredients List:** The ingredients are listed in descending order by weight. Choose products with a short, recognizable ingredient list. Avoid items with added sugars, trans fats, and artificial additives.
- **Nutritional Information:** Pay attention to serving sizes, as the nutritional information is based on a specific portion. Check the amounts of calories, fats, sugars, sodium, and fiber.
- **Whole Foods:** Focus on whole, minimally processed foods that provide essential nutrients without added sugars or unhealthy fats.
  - **Examples:** Fresh fruits and vegetables, whole grains, lean proteins, and healthy fats.

**Tips for Budget-Friendly Healthy Shopping**

Eating healthy doesn't have to be expensive. Here are some tips to help you shop for nutritious foods on a budget:

- **Plan Your Meals:** As mentioned in the meal planning section, having a plan helps you avoid impulse buys and ensures you only purchase what you need.
- **Buy in Bulk:** Purchase staples like grains, beans, and nuts in bulk to save money. These items have a long shelf life and can be used in a variety of meals.
- **Choose Seasonal Produce:** Fruits and vegetables are often cheaper and fresher when they're in season. Consider visiting local farmers' markets for deals.
- **Use Store Brands:** Store-brand items are often less expensive than name brands and can be just as nutritious.
- **Minimize Processed Foods:** Processed foods are often more expensive and less nutritious. Focus on whole foods, which are typically more budget-friendly and better for your health.
- **Frozen and Canned Options:** Frozen fruits and vegetables are often more affordable and just as nutritious as fresh. Choose canned goods without added sugars or sodium.

By making strategic choices at the grocery store, you can eat healthily without breaking the bank.

**6.4 Cooking Healthy Meals at Home**

Cooking at home allows you to control what goes into your food and make healthier choices. Simple cooking techniques and healthy recipes can help you prepare delicious meals that support your dietary goals.

**Simple and Healthy Recipes**

Here are some ideas for simple, nutritious meals you can prepare at home:

- **Vegetable Stir-Fry:** Sauté a variety of vegetables like bell peppers, broccoli, carrots, and snap peas in a small amount of olive oil. Add a lean protein like chicken, tofu, or shrimp, and serve over brown rice or quinoa.
- **Baked Salmon with Asparagus:** Season a salmon fillet with lemon, garlic, and herbs, and bake alongside asparagus spears. Serve with a side of roasted sweet potatoes.
- **Quinoa Salad:** Cook quinoa and toss it with chopped vegetables, such as cucumber, tomato, and bell pepper. Add chickpeas for protein, and dress with olive oil, lemon juice, and fresh herbs.
- **Lentil Soup:** Simmer lentils with diced tomatoes, carrots, celery, onion, and garlic in vegetable broth. Season with cumin, turmeric, and coriander for a warming, nutrient-dense soup.
- **Overnight Oats:** Mix rolled oats with almond milk, chia seeds, and a touch of honey. Let it sit overnight in the fridge, then top with fresh berries and nuts in the morning.

**Techniques for Reducing Fat, Sugar, and Salt**

Making small changes in how you cook can significantly reduce the amount of fat, sugar, and salt in your meals:

- **Use Healthy Fats:** Replace butter with olive oil or avocado oil for cooking. These oils contain heart-healthy monounsaturated fats.
- **Reduce Sugar:** Use natural sweeteners like honey, maple syrup, or mashed bananas instead of refined sugar. You can also reduce the amount of sugar in recipes by half without compromising flavor.
- **Limit Salt:** Enhance the flavor of your dishes with herbs, spices, lemon juice, or vinegar instead of salt. If you use salt, opt for sea salt or kosher salt, and add it sparingly.
- **Steam or Grill:** Steam vegetables or grill proteins instead of frying to reduce added fats.
- **Bulk Up with Vegetables:** Add more vegetables to dishes like pasta, casseroles, and soups to increase fiber and nutrients while reducing calorie density.

Cooking at home with these techniques can help you create meals that are both healthy and satisfying.

### 6.5 Eating Out and Maintaining a Healthy Diet

Eating out can be challenging when trying to stick to a healthy diet, but with a few strategies, you can make better choices and enjoy meals out without compromising your health goals.

**How to Make Healthy Choices at Restaurants**

When dining out, consider the following tips to make healthier choices:

- **Research Menus in Advance:** Many restaurants post their menus online. Reviewing the menu ahead of time can help you make a healthier choice before you arrive.
- **Ask for Modifications:** Don't be afraid to ask for changes to your order, such as grilling instead of frying, dressing on the side, or substituting a salad for fries.
- **Portion Control:** Restaurant portions are often larger than necessary. Consider sharing a dish, ordering an appetizer as your main course, or taking half of your meal home.
- **Focus on Veggies:** Look for dishes that emphasize vegetables, such as salads, stir-fries, or vegetable-based soups. You can also ask for extra vegetables on the side.
- **Choose Lean Proteins:** Opt for grilled, baked, or steamed proteins like chicken, fish, or tofu rather than fried or breaded options.
- **Limit Sauces and Dressings:** Sauces and dressings can add extra calories, sugar, and sodium. Ask for them on the side and use them sparingly.

**Dealing with Social Situations and Peer Pressure**

Social situations can present challenges when trying to maintain a healthy diet. Here's how to handle them:

- **Communicate Your Goals:** Let friends and family know about your dietary goals. They are more likely to support you if they understand your commitment to a healthy lifestyle.
- **Offer to Bring a Dish:** If you're attending a potluck or family gathering, bring a healthy dish that you enjoy and that aligns with your dietary goals.
- **Practice Mindful Eating:** In social situations, it's easy to overeat. Pay attention to your hunger cues, eat slowly, and savor each bite.
- **Plan Ahead:** If you know you'll be attending an event with limited healthy options, eat a small, healthy meal beforehand to avoid overeating.
- **Set Boundaries:** It's okay to politely decline food or drinks that don't fit your dietary plan. You can also use strategies like taking small portions or choosing healthier options.

By being mindful of your choices and planning ahead, you can enjoy eating out and social events while staying true to your healthy diet.

# Conclusion

### 7.1 Summary of Key Points

Throughout this guide, we have explored the critical role that diet plays in overall health and well-being. We began by understanding the fundamental science of nutrition, including the importance of macronutrients, micronutrients, and hydration. We then delved into various popular diets, examining their benefits, potential risks, and suitability for different individuals.

Key points from each chapter include:

- **The Science of Nutrition:** Understanding the balance of carbohydrates, proteins, fats, vitamins, and minerals is essential for maintaining optimal health. Water and hydration are equally important, supporting every bodily function.
- **Popular Diet Types:** Different diets, such as the Mediterranean, Ketogenic, and Plant-Based diets, offer various health benefits. Choosing the right diet depends on individual health goals, lifestyle, and preferences.
- **Diet for Specific Health Goals:** Whether aiming for weight loss, muscle gain, cardiovascular health, or mental well-being, tailoring your diet to meet specific objectives is crucial. Each health goal requires a different focus on nutrients and dietary strategies.
- **Tailoring Diets to Different Life Stages:** Nutritional needs change throughout life, from childhood to old age. Understanding and adapting your diet to these changes can help maintain health and prevent disease.
- **Addressing Specific Health Conditions:** For conditions like diabetes, hypertension, autoimmune diseases, cancer, and osteoporosis, diet plays a vital role in management and prevention. Specific dietary adjustments can significantly impact health outcomes.
- **Practical Steps to Implementing a Healthy Diet:** Setting realistic goals, meal planning, smart grocery shopping, cooking at home, and making healthy choices when eating out are practical ways to maintain a healthy diet and achieve your health goals.

By understanding these key concepts, you are better equipped to make informed dietary choices that align with your personal health goals.

## 7.2 The Future of Diet and Nutrition

The field of diet and nutrition is continually evolving, with new research and technologies emerging that offer deeper insights into how food impacts our health. Some of the trends shaping the future of diet and nutrition include:

- **Personalized Nutrition:** Advances in genetic testing and microbiome analysis are paving the way for personalized nutrition plans tailored to an individual's unique genetic makeup and gut flora. This approach aims to optimize health outcomes by aligning diet with an individual's specific needs.
- **Plant-Based Eating:** As environmental and ethical concerns grow, more people are turning to plant-based diets. The rise of plant-based meat alternatives and increased

awareness of the benefits of reducing meat consumption are likely to continue shaping dietary habits.

- **Sustainability:** The focus on sustainable eating practices, such as choosing locally sourced, organic, and eco-friendly foods, is becoming increasingly important. This trend reflects a broader awareness of the environmental impact of food choices.
- **Technology and Diet Tracking:** Wearable technology and mobile apps that track dietary intake, physical activity, and other health metrics are becoming more sophisticated. These tools help individuals monitor their diet and make adjustments in real-time, promoting healthier habits.
- **Functional Foods:** The demand for functional foods—foods that provide health benefits beyond basic nutrition, such as probiotics, prebiotics, and superfoods—is on the rise. These foods are being incorporated into daily diets to support specific health goals.

As these trends develop, staying informed and adaptable will be crucial to making the best dietary choices for your health and the health of the planet.

**7.3 Final Thoughts**

Achieving and maintaining a healthy diet is a lifelong journey that requires knowledge, commitment, and flexibility. There is no one-size-fits-all approach to nutrition; the best diet is one that meets your individual needs, fits into your lifestyle, and is sustainable over the long term.

Remember, a healthy diet is about balance and enjoyment. It's not about strict limitations or deprivation, but rather making informed choices that contribute to your overall well-being. It's also important to be kind to yourself—making small, gradual changes is often more effective and sustainable than attempting drastic overhauls.

As you move forward on your journey to better health, use the information in this guide as a foundation to build a diet that supports your goals and enriches your life. Stay curious, stay informed, and above all, listen to your body's needs.

Thank you for taking the time to explore this guide. Here's to your health and well-being!

www.ingramcontent.com/pod-product-compliance
Lightning Source LLC
Chambersburg PA
CBHW081827250726
48657CB00011B/3511